CKD STAGE 4 COOKBOOK FOR SENIORS

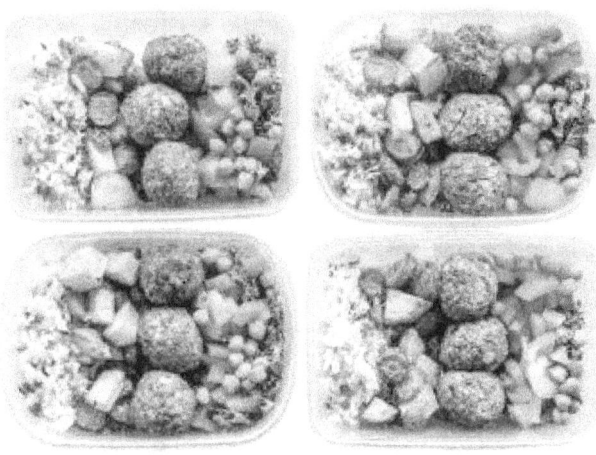

DR. JESSICA SMITH

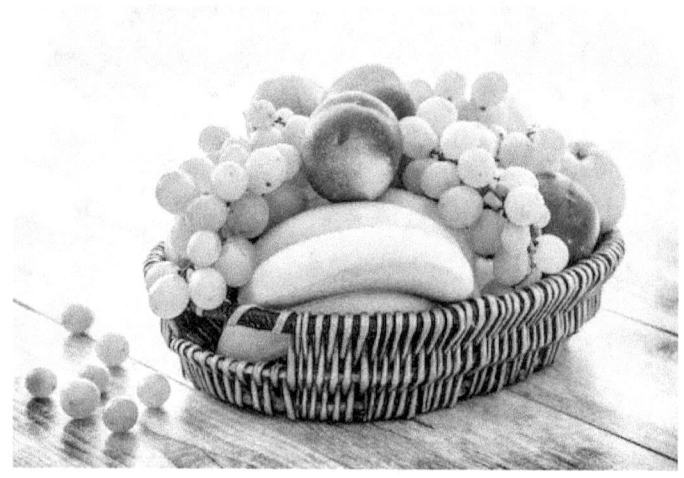

TABLE OF CONTENT

5

INTRODUCTION TO CHRONIC KIDNEY DISEASE

Introduction to Chronic Kidney Disease (CKD) marks the beginning of a transformative journey in the realm of health. As the kidneys, the unsung heroes of our internal ecosystem, face challenges, the repercussions resonate throughout the body. CKD is a progressive condition that necessitates a nuanced understanding to navigate its complexities.

At its core, CKD involves the gradual loss of kidney function over time. These vital organs, resembling sophisticated filtration systems, play a pivotal role in maintaining the delicate balance of fluids, electrolytes, and waste products within our bodies. The onset of CKD triggers a cascade of physiological changes, challenging the body's homeostasis.

The journey into CKD typically unfolds in stages, each marked by a distinct degree of kidney impairment. Understanding these stages is crucial in gauging the severity of the condition and tailoring appropriate interventions. From the early stages, where symptoms may be subtle, to the advanced stages, where the impact on overall health becomes more pronounced, CKD demands a comprehensive grasp.

Beyond the physical dimensions, CKD is often intertwined with various risk factors, ranging from genetic predispositions to lifestyle choices.

Age, diabetes, hypertension, and certain medications can contribute to the onset and progression of CKD. Recognizing these factors is instrumental in both prevention and management.

This introduction serves as a gateway to a deeper exploration of CKD, setting the stage for unraveling the intricacies of this condition.

As we delve into the subsequent chapters, we embark on a quest for knowledge that empowers individuals, caregivers, and healthcare professionals alike to navigate the challenges posed by Chronic Kidney Disease with resilience and understanding.

CHAPTER ONE

Definition and Stages

Chronic Kidney Disease (CKD) is a multifaceted condition characterized by the gradual deterioration of kidney function over an extended period. Understanding its definition and the distinct stages through which it progresses is foundational to addressing the complexities of this pervasive health challenge.

Definition of Chronic Kidney Disease:

CKD is not a singular disease but rather a term that encapsulates a spectrum of renal disorders resulting in prolonged damage to the kidneys.

These vital organs, resembling intricate filters, play a crucial role in maintaining the body's internal equilibrium. CKD disrupts this delicate balance, leading to an accumulation of waste products, electrolyte imbalances, and compromised fluid regulation.

The hallmark of CKD is the persistence of kidney damage or a decline in kidney function for three months or more. This impairment is often accompanied by structural abnormalities and abnormalities in urine composition. The etiology of CKD is diverse, encompassing conditions such as diabetes, hypertension, glomerulonephritis, and polycystic kidney disease. Recognizing and diagnosing CKD early is imperative for implementing effective interventions that can slow its progression and mitigate associated complications.

Stages of Chronic Kidney Disease:

CKD is stratified into stages based on the Glomerular Filtration Rate (GFR), a measure of how efficiently the kidneys filter waste from the blood. The National Kidney Foundation defines five stages:

Stage 1 (GFR > 90 mL/min): Kidney damage with normal or increased GFR. This stage often exhibits few, if any, symptoms, making early detection challenging.

Stage 2 (GFR 60-89 mL/min): Mild reduction in kidney function. As GFR decreases, the risk of complications and progression to advanced stages rises.

Stage 3 (GFR 30-59 mL/min): Moderate reduction in kidney function. Symptoms may become more noticeable, and interventions to manage underlying causes become crucial.

Stage 4 (GFR 15-29 mL/min): Severe reduction in kidney function. The risk of complications, including cardiovascular issues and anemia, intensifies. Comprehensive management strategies are essential at this stage.

Stage 5 (GFR < 15 mL/min): End-Stage Renal Disease (ESRD). Kidney function is significantly impaired, necessitating renal replacement therapy such as dialysis or kidney transplantation for survival.

Understanding the stages of CKD is pivotal for healthcare professionals to tailor interventions, monitor progression, and educate individuals about lifestyle modifications.

Early detection and management can significantly improve outcomes and enhance the quality of life for those navigating the challenges of chronic kidney disease.

Prevalence in Seniors

The prevalence of Chronic Kidney Disease (CKD) in seniors is a pressing health concern, underscoring the intersection of aging and the vulnerability of vital organ function. As individuals gracefully traverse the later stages of life, the kidneys, the unassuming heroes of the body's filtration system, often bear the brunt of time, contributing to a heightened prevalence of CKD among the elderly.

The Aging Paradox:

Aging, a natural and inevitable process, intricately intertwines with the prevalence of CKD in seniors. The kidneys undergo structural and functional changes over time, experiencing a gradual decline in mass and efficiency.

The number of functioning nephrons, the microscopic units responsible for filtering blood, decreases, compromising the kidneys' ability to regulate fluid balance and eliminate waste products.

Prevalence Rates:

Epidemiological studies consistently highlight a rising prevalence of CKD with advancing age. The risk of developing CKD increases exponentially in the senior population, with a substantial proportion facing the challenges of impaired renal function.

Factors such as reduced renal blood flow, diminished nephron function, and age-related vascular changes contribute to this heightened vulnerability.

Moreover, the aging process often converges with other risk factors for CKD, such as hypertension and diabetes, further amplifying the prevalence among seniors. Chronic conditions prevalent in older adults can instigate and exacerbate kidney damage, creating a complex interplay of health dynamics.

Impact on Health Outcomes:

The implications of CKD in seniors extend beyond the confines of renal function, influencing overall health outcomes. Seniors with CKD face an increased risk of cardiovascular complications, anemia, and frailty.

Additionally, the presence of CKD can complicate the management of other chronic conditions, requiring a comprehensive and tailored approach to healthcare in the elderly population.

Recognizing the prevalence of CKD in seniors is a crucial step toward implementing proactive measures. Routine screenings and early detection can facilitate timely interventions to slow the progression of CKD and alleviate associated complications.

Moreover, understanding the unique challenges faced by seniors with CKD allows healthcare providers to customize treatment plans, considering factors such as medication management, dietary adjustments, and lifestyle modifications that align with the aging process.

Overview of CKD Stage 4

Navigating the terrain of Chronic Kidney Disease (CKD) Stage 4 represents a critical juncture in the continuum of renal health. As the kidneys, those intricate filtration marvels, confront significant impairment, an overview of CKD Stage 4 becomes imperative for comprehending the nuanced challenges and formulating effective management strategies.

Defining CKD Stage 4:

CKD Stage 4 is characterized by a substantial decline in kidney function, as measured by the Glomerular Filtration Rate (GFR). At this stage, the GFR typically falls within the range of 15 to 29 milliliters per minute, signifying severe impairment.

The kidneys' ability to filter blood, regulate fluid balance, and excrete waste products is significantly compromised, elevating the risk of complications and necessitating vigilant medical attention.

Common Symptoms:

The journey through CKD Stage 4 is often accompanied by a constellation of symptoms. Fatigue, persistent fluid retention leading to swelling (edema), increased blood pressure, and electrolyte imbalances are among the notable indicators.

Individuals may also experience changes in urinary patterns, with alterations in frequency and volume. Anemia, a common consequence of impaired kidney function, can manifest, contributing to further fatigue and diminished well-being.

Risk of Complications:

CKD Stage 4 elevates the risk of various complications, extending beyond renal challenges. Cardiovascular issues become pronounced, with an increased susceptibility to heart disease and related complications. Anemia, a result of reduced erythropoietin production by the kidneys, poses additional health concerns.

Bone health may be compromised due to imbalances in calcium and phosphorus levels, contributing to renal osteodystrophy.

Management Strategies:

Effectively navigating CKD Stage 4 involves a comprehensive and multidisciplinary approach. Renal specialists collaborate with healthcare teams to address underlying causes and manage symptoms. Lifestyle modifications, including dietary changes to regulate fluid and electrolyte intake, become paramount. Medications are often prescribed to manage blood pressure, treat anemia, and mitigate complications.

Preparing for Advanced Care:

As individuals traverse CKD Stage 4, discussions surrounding advanced care planning become integral. Exploring renal replacement therapies, such as dialysis or kidney transplantation, becomes crucial for those approaching End-Stage Renal Disease (ESRD).

Healthcare providers work collaboratively with patients and their families to make informed decisions aligned with individual values and preferences.

Identifying Stage 4

Identifying Chronic Kidney Disease (CKD) Stage 4 is a pivotal step in the proactive management of renal health. As the condition progresses to this advanced stage, early detection becomes paramount for implementing targeted interventions and mitigating the risk of complications.

Recognizing the distinctive markers and employing diagnostic tools are essential components in the journey of identifying CKD Stage 4.

Clinical Markers:

Clinical indicators play a crucial role in identifying CKD Stage 4. Symptoms may become more pronounced at this stage, prompting individuals and healthcare providers to delve deeper into the underlying causes.

Fatigue, persistent edema, changes in urinary habits, and elevated blood pressure are common manifestations. Anemia, often associated with impaired kidney function, may contribute to a sense of lethargy and weakness.

Laboratory Tests:

Laboratory tests serve as invaluable tools in the identification of CKD Stage 4. The Glomerular Filtration Rate (GFR), a measure of kidney function, is a key parameter. In Sta

ge 4, the GFR typically falls within the range of 15 to 29 milliliters per minute, indicating a severe decline. Blood tests assess creatinine and urea levels, providing insights into the kidneys' ability to filter waste products. Elevated levels of these substances may signal impaired renal function.

Imaging Studies:

Imaging studies, such as ultrasounds and CT scans, contribute to the identification process by offering a visual assessment of the kidneys' structure and detecting any abnormalities. These studies can reveal the presence of cysts, tumors, or other structural issues that may contribute to or result from CKD Stage 4.

Biopsy:

In certain cases, a kidney biopsy may be recommended to confirm the diagnosis and assess the extent of kidney damage. This invasive procedure involves extracting a small sample of kidney tissue for microscopic examination. Biopsies can provide crucial information about the underlying causes of CKD and guide treatment decisions.

Regular Monitoring:

Identifying CKD Stage 4 is not a one-time event; it necessitates ongoing monitoring, especially for individuals at higher risk or those with underlying conditions like diabetes or hypertension.

Regular check-ups, including blood pressure measurements and laboratory tests, enable healthcare providers to track changes in kidney function and adjust management strategies accordingly.

Multidisciplinary Collaboration:

A collaborative approach involving healthcare providers from various specialties is integral to the identification and management of CKD Stage 4. Nephrologists, primary care physicians, and other specialists work in tandem to interpret clinical findings, tailor treatment plans, and address comorbidities that may exacerbate kidney impairment.

Common Symptoms and Signs

Common symptoms and signs play a crucial role in identifying and understanding Chronic Kidney Disease (CKD) Stage 4, marking a significant stage in the continuum of renal health.

As kidney function becomes severely impaired, a spectrum of manifestations emerges, guiding individuals and healthcare providers in recognizing and addressing the challenges presented by CKD at this advanced stage.

1. Fatigue and Weakness:

Fatigue is a hallmark symptom of CKD Stage 4, often attributed to anemia resulting from diminished erythropoietin production by the kidneys.

The decrease in oxygen-carrying red blood cells can lead to a sense of weakness, exhaustion, and reduced stamina, impacting the overall quality of life for individuals navigating this stage.

2. Edema (Swelling):

Persistent fluid retention, known as edema, is a common sign of impaired kidney function.

As the kidneys struggle to regulate fluid balance, excess fluid can accumulate in the body, particularly in the ankles, legs, and around the eyes. Edema can contribute to discomfort and pose challenges in daily activities.

3. Changes in Urinary Patterns:

Altered urinary habits are characteristic of CKD Stage 4. Individuals may experience changes in frequency, urgency, or volume of urine output.

Additionally, foamy or bubbly urine may indicate the presence of protein, a key marker of kidney damage. These changes underscore the kidneys' struggle to maintain proper filtration and waste elimination.

4. Elevated Blood Pressure:

Hypertension is both a cause and a consequence of CKD. In Stage 4, elevated blood pressure becomes more prevalent and is often challenging to control.

The intricate relationship between kidney function and blood pressure regulation underscores the bidirectional impact of these factors on one another.

5. Shortness of Breath:

As CKD progresses to Stage 4, the accumulation of waste products in the body can lead to respiratory challenges. Shortness of breath may result from fluid overload, anemia, or cardiovascular complications associated with advanced kidney impairment.

6. Anemia:

Anemia is a common complication of CKD Stage 4, arising from the kidneys' reduced ability to produce erythropoietin, a hormone crucial for red blood cell production. Fatigue, weakness, and pallor are characteristic of anemia, highlighting the intricate connections between kidney function and overall blood health.

7. Cognitive Impairment:

In some cases, CKD Stage 4 may manifest with cognitive changes. Individuals may experience difficulty concentrating, memory lapses, or mental fog.

These cognitive impairments can be attributed to factors such as anemia, fluid imbalances, and the cumulative impact of chronic illness on overall well-being.

8. Bone and Joint Problems:

Imbalances in calcium and phosphorus levels associated with CKD can affect bone health. Individuals may experience bone pain, fractures, or joint discomfort, collectively referred to as renal osteodystrophy. These musculoskeletal issues add to the complexity of symptoms in CKD Stage 4.

Recognizing these common symptoms and signs is pivotal for timely intervention and tailored management strategies. As CKD Stage 4 poses multifaceted challenges, a comprehensive approach involving healthcare providers, specialists, and individuals themselves is crucial in addressing the nuanced manifestations and enhancing the quality of life for those navigating this advanced stage of chronic kidney disease.

Causes of Chronic Kidney Disease (CKD) Stage 4:

CKD Stage 4 is often the result of a complex interplay of factors, each contributing to the progressive decline in kidney function. The primary causes include:

Hypertension (High Blood Pressure): Prolonged, uncontrolled hypertension is a leading cause of CKD. The constant strain on the blood vessels in the kidneys can result in damage to the nephrons, impairing their ability to filter blood effectively.

Diabetes Mellitus: Diabetes is a significant contributor to CKD Stage 4. Elevated blood sugar levels over time can damage the small blood vessels in the kidneys, leading to diabetic nephropathy. This condition accelerates the progression of CKD, particularly in individuals with poorly controlled diabetes.

Glomerulonephritis: Inflammation of the glomeruli, the filtering units of the kidneys, can result in glomerulonephritis. This inflammatory process can be caused by infections, autoimmune disorders, or other immune system abnormalities, leading to structural damage in the kidneys.

Polycystic Kidney Disease (PKD): A genetic disorder, PKD leads to the formation of fluid-filled cysts in the kidneys.

These cysts gradually replace normal kidney tissue, compromising function. As PKD progresses, it can contribute to the development of CKD Stage 4.

Obstructive Disorders: Conditions that obstruct the flow of urine, such as kidney stones, tumors, or an enlarged prostate, can cause kidney damage. The obstruction disrupts the normal flow of urine and, if left untreated, can lead to significant impairment in kidney function.

Vascular Disorders: Conditions affecting the blood vessels, such as renal artery stenosis or thrombosis, can compromise blood flow to the kidneys, contributing to CKD Stage 4.

Understanding the specific causes of CKD Stage 4 is essential for targeted interventions and management strategies. Addressing the underlying cause is pivotal in slowing the progression of kidney damage and improving overall outcomes.

Risk Factors for CKD Stage 4:

Several risk factors heighten the likelihood of developing CKD Stage 4. These include:

> ➤ Age: The risk of CKD increases with age, particularly in individuals over 60 years old.
> ➤ Family History: A genetic predisposition to kidney disease can elevate the risk. Conditions like PKD may run in families.
> ➤ Gender: Men are generally at a higher risk of developing CKD than women.

➢ Race and Ethnicity: Certain racial and ethnic groups, such as African Americans, Hispanics, and Native Americans, are at an increased risk of CKD.

➢ Smoking: Tobacco use can accelerate the progression of CKD, particularly in individuals with pre-existing kidney conditions.

➢ Cardiovascular Disease: Conditions like heart disease and stroke can contribute to kidney damage, and individuals with cardiovascular issues are at an elevated risk of CKD.

➢ Obesity: Excess body weight is associated with an increased risk of developing CKD, as it contributes to conditions like diabetes and hypertension.

➢ Existing Health Conditions: Chronic conditions such as hypertension, diabetes, and autoimmune disorders can significantly elevate the risk of CKD Stage 4.

Understanding these risk factors enables healthcare providers to identify individuals at higher risk and implement preventive measures and early interventions to mitigate the progression of CKD Stage 4.

CHAPTER TWO

Aging and Kidney Health

Aging is a natural and inevitable process that intricately intersects with kidney health, bringing about notable changes in the structure and function of these vital organs. Understanding the dynamics between aging and kidney health is essential as individuals progress through the later stages of life.

As individuals age, the kidneys undergo physiological alterations that contribute to a decline in their overall function. The number of nephrons, the microscopic units responsible for filtering blood and removing waste products, decreases with age.

This reduction in nephron count diminishes the kidneys' filtration capacity, impacting their ability to maintain fluid balance, regulate electrolytes, and eliminate toxins from the bloodstream.

The aging process also affects the blood vessels supplying the kidneys, leading to changes in renal blood flow. Reduced blood flow to the kidneys compromises their efficiency in filtering and processing blood, further contributing to age-related declines in kidney function.

While aging alone does not guarantee the development of kidney disease, it does render the kidneys more susceptible to the impact of other age-related conditions. Chronic conditions such as hypertension and diabetes, prevalent in older adults, can accelerate kidney damage and elevate the risk of developing chronic kidney disease (CKD).

Moreover, medications commonly prescribed for age-related conditions may have nephrotoxic effects, potentially exacerbating kidney dysfunction. Close monitoring and periodic assessments become crucial to ensure that medications are administered at optimal dosages, mitigating the risk of adverse effects on kidney health.

Despite these challenges, adopting a proactive approach to kidney health in the aging population is vital. Lifestyle modifications, including a well-balanced diet, regular exercise, and adequate hydration, play a pivotal role in supporting kidney function. Routine health check-ups that include assessments of blood pressure, blood glucose levels, and kidney function tests allow for early detection and intervention.

Aging and kidney health are intricately linked, with the aging process contributing to physiological changes that can impact renal function.

Awareness of these dynamics underscores the importance of proactive measures to promote kidney health in the elderly. As the population ages, fostering a holistic approach that integrates lifestyle modifications and regular health assessments becomes paramount in preserving and enhancing the well-being of the aging kidneys.

Contributing Medical Conditions

Contributing medical conditions play a significant role in the development and progression of Chronic Kidney Disease (CKD) Stage 4, amplifying the complexity of kidney health management.

Understanding the interconnectedness between CKD and these medical conditions is crucial for tailoring effective interventions and mitigating the impact on renal function.

Hypertension (High Blood Pressure): Hypertension is both a cause and a consequence of CKD Stage 4. The relentless strain on the blood vessels within the kidneys due to high blood pressure contributes to kidney damage over time. Conversely, impaired kidney function can lead to difficulty regulating blood pressure, creating a reciprocal relationship.

Diabetes Mellitus: Diabetes, particularly Type 2 diabetes, is a leading contributor to CKD Stage 4. Prolonged elevated blood sugar levels damage the delicate blood vessels and nephrons within the kidneys, accelerating the progression of kidney disease. Individuals with diabetes require vigilant management to mitigate the risk of CKD.

Cardiovascular Disease: Conditions such as heart disease and congestive heart failure significantly impact kidney health.

Reduced cardiac function can compromise blood flow to the kidneys, contributing to impaired filtration and worsening kidney function. Simultaneously, CKD increases the risk of cardiovascular complications, creating a symbiotic relationship.

Autoimmune Disorders: Certain autoimmune conditions, such as lupus and vasculitis, can target the kidneys, leading to inflammation and damage. Autoimmune-induced kidney diseases contribute to the complexity of managing CKD Stage 4, often requiring specialized treatment approaches.

Chronic Urinary Tract Infections (UTIs): Recurrent UTIs can lead to kidney damage, especially if left untreated. The persistent infection and inflammation compromise the structural integrity of the kidneys, contributing to the progression of CKD.

Polycystic Kidney Disease (PKD): A genetic disorder, PKD leads to the formation of fluid-filled cysts within the kidneys. These cysts gradually replace healthy tissue, impairing kidney function. PKD is a significant contributing factor to the development of CKD Stage 4.

Obesity: Excess body weight is associated with an increased risk of developing CKD, as it often contributes to conditions like diabetes and hypertension.

Obesity-related metabolic changes can further impact renal function, creating a milieu conducive to kidney disease.

Aging: While not a medical condition per se, aging is a significant contributing factor to CKD Stage 4. The natural aging process brings about structural and functional changes in the kidneys, rendering them more vulnerable to the impact of other medical conditions and exacerbating the progression of CKD.

Addressing contributing medical conditions in the context of CKD Stage 4 requires a comprehensive and multidisciplinary approach. Healthcare providers collaborate to manage not only the kidney disease but also the interconnected web of conditions that influence its trajectory, emphasizing the importance of holistic patient care in navigating the challenges posed by advanced kidney impairment.

Genetic Factors

Genetic factors play a crucial role in shaping the landscape of Chronic Kidney Disease (CKD) Stage 4, underscoring the intricate interplay between inherited traits and renal health. Understanding the genetic underpinnings of kidney disease is instrumental in unraveling its complexities and tailoring interventions for individuals with a hereditary predisposition.

Polycystic Kidney Disease (PKD): One of the most prominent genetic contributors to CKD Stage 4 is Polycystic Kidney Disease. Autosomal Dominant Polycystic Kidney Disease (ADPKD) and Autosomal Recessive Polycystic Kidney Disease (ARPKD) are inherited conditions characterized by the formation of fluid-filled cysts in the kidneys. These cysts gradually replace healthy kidney tissue, compromising function and leading to the progression of CKD.

Alport Syndrome: This genetic disorder affects the glomerular basement membrane in the kidneys. It is characterized by kidney inflammation, hematuria (blood in urine), and can progress to CKD. Alport Syndrome can be inherited in an X-linked recessive, autosomal recessive, or autosomal dominant manner.

Hereditary Nephritis: Certain forms of hereditary nephritis, also known as familial glomerulonephritis, are linked to genetic mutations affecting the glomeruli.

These mutations can result in inflammation and scarring, contributing to the development of CKD.

Genetic Predisposition to Hypertension and Diabetes: Genetic factors can influence an individual's susceptibility to conditions like hypertension and Type 2 diabetes, both of which are major risk factors for CKD.

Inherited traits may impact blood pressure regulation, insulin sensitivity, and other factors that contribute to the development of these conditions.

Familial Clustering of Kidney Disease: In some cases, a family history of kidney disease itself can be a genetic factor. While specific genetic mutations may not be identified, the aggregation of renal conditions within families suggests a potential genetic predisposition.

Understanding the genetic factors associated with CKD Stage 4 is vital for risk assessment, early detection, and personalized management strategies. Genetic testing, when available and appropriate, can help identify individuals at higher risk due to inherited conditions, enabling healthcare providers to implement preventive measures and closely monitor kidney health.

The evolving field of genetic medicine holds promise for uncovering new insights into the genetic basis of kidney disease, paving the way for more targeted and precise interventions in the realm of renal health.

Foods to eat and Avoid

Foods to Eat for CKD Stage 4:

Low-Potassium Fruits: Opt for fruits with lower potassium content, such as apples, berries, and grapes. These choices help maintain potassium balance in individuals with compromised kidney function.

Low-Phosphorus Foods: Incorporate foods low in phosphorus, including green beans, peppers, and cabbage. Managing phosphorus intake is crucial to prevent complications associated with elevated phosphorus levels in CKD Stage 4.

Lean Proteins: Choose lean protein sources like skinless poultry, fish, and tofu. Adequate protein intake is essential, and opting for lean sources helps manage protein levels without overburdening the kidneys.

Whole Grains: Embrace whole grains like brown rice, quinoa, and whole wheat bread. These provide essential nutrients and fiber without contributing excessive amounts of phosphorus.

Vegetables with Low Potassium: Include vegetables with lower potassium levels, such as cucumbers, carrots, and lettuce. Balancing potassium intake is crucial in supporting kidney function.

Foods to Avoid for CKD Stage 4:

High-Potassium Foods: Limit high-potassium foods, including bananas, oranges, and potatoes. Elevated potassium levels can pose risks for individuals with compromised kidney function.

Phosphorus-Rich Foods: Restrict phosphorus-rich foods such as dairy products, nuts, and processed foods. Excessive phosphorus intake can contribute to mineral imbalances in CKD Stage 4.

Processed and Packaged Foods: Minimize the consumption of processed and packaged foods, as they often contain hidden salts, additives, and phosphorus additives that can strain the kidneys.

Red and Processed Meats: Cut back on red and processed meats, as they can contribute to protein breakdown and increase the burden on the kidneys.

High-Sodium Foods: Reduce sodium intake by avoiding highly salted foods like processed snacks, canned soups, and certain condiments. Managing sodium helps control blood pressure and fluid balance in CKD Stage 4.

7-day meal plan for Ckd Stage Stage 4 For Seniors

Day 1: Grilled Lemon Herb Chicken with Quinoa and Steamed Vegetables

Ingredients:

Boneless, skinless chicken breasts

Lemon

Fresh herbs (such as rosemary, thyme, and parsley)

Quinoa

Mixed vegetables (carrots, green beans, and zucchini)

Instructions:

Marinate chicken with lemon juice, chopped herbs, salt, and pepper.

Grill the chicken until fully cooked.

Prepare quinoa according to package instructions.

Steam mixed vegetables until tender.

Serve grilled chicken over a bed of quinoa with steamed vegetables on the side.

Day 2: Baked Salmon with Sweet Potato and Asparagus

Ingredients:

Salmon fillets

Sweet potatoes

Asparagus spears

Olive oil

Garlic powder

Lemon zest

Instructions:

Preheat the oven and line a baking sheet.

Season salmon with garlic powder, lemon zest, salt, and pepper.

Place salmon on the baking sheet alongside sliced sweet potatoes and asparagus.

Drizzle with olive oil and bake until the salmon is cooked through.

Serve the baked salmon with roasted sweet potatoes and asparagus.

Day 3: Lentil Soup with Whole Grain Toast

Ingredients:

Dry lentils

Carrots

Celery

Onion

Low-sodium vegetable broth

Whole grain bread

Instructions:

Rinse lentils and combine with chopped vegetables in a pot.

Add low-sodium vegetable broth and bring to a boil.

Simmer until lentils are tender and vegetables are cooked.

Toast whole grain bread slices.

Serve lentil soup with a side of whole grain toast.

Day 4: Stir-Fried Tofu with Brown Rice and Broccoli

Ingredients:

Extra-firm tofu

Brown rice

Broccoli florets

Low-sodium soy sauce

Ginger

Garlic

Sesame oil

Instructions:

Press and cube tofu.

Cook brown rice according to package instructions.

Stir-fry tofu in sesame oil with minced ginger and garlic.

Add broccoli and soy sauce, cooking until vegetables are tender.

Serve stir-fried tofu and broccoli over cooked brown rice.

Day 5: Chicken and Vegetable Skewers with Quinoa Salad

Ingredients:

Chicken thighs, cut into chunks

Bell peppers (various colors)

Cherry tomatoes

Red onion

Quinoa

Cucumber

Feta cheese

Olive oil and balsamic vinegar for dressing

Instructions:

Thread chicken and vegetables onto skewers.

Grill until chicken is fully cooked.

Prepare quinoa and let it cool.

Mix quinoa with diced cucumber, cherry tomatoes, and crumbled feta.

Serve chicken and vegetable skewers on a bed of quinoa salad.

Day 6: Shrimp Stir-Fry with Brown Rice

Ingredients:

Shrimp, peeled and deveined

Brown rice

Mixed stir-fry vegetables (bell peppers, snap peas, carrots)

Low-sodium teriyaki sauce

Olive oil

Sesame seeds for garnish

Instructions:

Cook brown rice according to package instructions.

Stir-fry shrimp and vegetables in olive oil.

Add low-sodium teriyaki sauce and cook until shrimp are pink.

Serve shrimp stir-fry over brown rice, garnished with sesame seeds.

Day 7: Vegetable and Chickpea Salad with Grilled Chicken

Ingredients:

Grilled chicken breast

Mixed salad greens

Cherry tomatoes

Cucumber

Red onion

Chickpeas (canned, drained)

Balsamic vinaigrette dressing

Instructions:

Grill chicken until fully cooked.

Assemble a salad with mixed greens, cherry tomatoes, sliced cucumber, red onion, and chickpeas.

Slice grilled chicken and place on top of the salad.

Drizzle with balsamic vinaigrette dressing.

Note: Before starting any new meal plan, it's essential for seniors with CKD Stage 4 to consult with their healthcare team or a registered dietitian to ensure the plan aligns with their individual dietary needs and restrictions. Adjust portion sizes based on individual requirements.

CHAPTER THREE

CKD Stage 4 Recipes for Seniors

Breakfast

1. Scrambled Egg Whites with Spinach and Toast

Ingredients:

Egg whites

Fresh spinach

Whole grain toast

Olive oil

Salt and pepper

Instructions:

Heat olive oil in a pan.

Add fresh spinach and sauté until wilted.

Pour in egg whites, season with salt and pepper, and scramble.

Serve over whole grain toast.

2. Blueberry Oatmeal

Ingredients:

Rolled oats

Fresh blueberries

Almond milk

Chia seeds

Cinnamon

Instructions:

Cook rolled oats with almond milk.

Stir in fresh blueberries, chia seeds, and a sprinkle of cinnamon.

Cook until oats are tender.

Serve warm.

3. Greek Yogurt Parfait with Berries

Ingredients:

Low-fat Greek yogurt

Strawberries, sliced

Raspberries

Granola (low in potassium)

Honey

Instructions:

Layer Greek yogurt with sliced strawberries and raspberries.

Top with low-potassium granola.

Drizzle with honey.

Enjoy the parfait.

4. Vegetable Omelette

Ingredients:

Eggs

Bell peppers (various colors)

Tomatoes

Onion

Low-fat cheese (optional)

Instructions:

Whisk eggs and pour into a non-stick pan.

Add diced bell peppers, tomatoes, and onions.

Cook until eggs are set.

Fold the omelette and, if desired, add low-fat cheese.

5. Cottage Cheese with Pineapple

Ingredients:

Low-fat cottage cheese

Fresh pineapple, diced

Instructions:

Combine cottage cheese with diced fresh pineapple.

Mix well.

Serve chilled.

6. Banana Nut Smoothie

Ingredients:

Banana

Almond milk

Low-potassium nut butter (almond or cashew)

Ice cubes

Instructions:

Blend banana, almond milk, nut butter, and ice cubes until smooth.

Pour into a glass.

Garnish with chopped nuts if desired.

7. Avocado Toast with Cherry Tomatoes

Ingredients:

Whole grain bread

Ripe avocado

Cherry tomatoes

Lemon juice

Olive oil

Salt and pepper

Instructions:

Toast whole grain bread.

Mash ripe avocado and spread over the toast.

Top with sliced cherry tomatoes.

Drizzle with lemon juice, olive oil, and season with salt and pepper.

8. Quinoa Breakfast Bowl

Ingredients:

Quinoa

Low-fat milk or almond milk

Sliced peaches

Cinnamon

Chopped nuts (almonds or walnuts)

Instructions:

Cook quinoa with low-fat milk.

Top with sliced peaches, a sprinkle of cinnamon, and chopped nuts.

Serve warm.

9. Apple Cinnamon Pancakes

Ingredients:

Whole grain pancake mix

Unsweetened applesauce

Cinnamon

Maple syrup (optional)

Instructions:

Prepare pancake mix according to package instructions.

Add unsweetened applesauce and cinnamon to the batter.

Cook pancakes on a griddle.

Serve with a drizzle of maple syrup if desired.

10. Spinach and Feta Breakfast Wrap

Ingredients:

Whole wheat tortilla

Egg whites

Fresh spinach

Feta cheese (low in sodium)

Cherry tomatoes, sliced

Instructions:

Scramble egg whites and cook in a pan.

Place cooked egg whites on a whole wheat tortilla.

Add fresh spinach, crumbled feta, and sliced cherry tomatoes.

Wrap and enjoy.

Lunch

1. Grilled Lemon Herb Salmon with Quinoa and Steamed Asparagus

Ingredients:

Salmon fillets

Lemon

Fresh herbs (rosemary, thyme, parsley)

Quinoa

Asparagus spears

Instructions:

Marinate salmon with lemon juice, chopped herbs, salt, and pepper.

Grill salmon until fully cooked.

Cook quinoa according to package instructions.

Steam asparagus until tender.

Serve grilled salmon over quinoa with steamed asparagus on the side.

2. Turkey and Vegetable Stir-Fry with Brown Rice

Ingredients:

Ground turkey

Mixed stir-fry vegetables (bell peppers, broccoli, carrots)

Low-sodium soy sauce

Brown rice

Instructions:

Cook ground turkey in a pan until browned.

Add mixed vegetables and stir-fry until tender.

Season with low-sodium soy sauce.

Cook brown rice according to package instructions.

Serve turkey and vegetable stir-fry over cooked brown rice.

3. Lentil and Vegetable Soup

Ingredients:

Dry lentils

Carrots

Celery

Onion

Low-sodium vegetable broth

Spinach leaves

Instructions:

Rinse lentils and combine with chopped vegetables in a pot.

Add low-sodium vegetable broth and bring to a boil.

Simmer until lentils are tender and vegetables are cooked.

Add spinach leaves and cook until wilted.

Serve warm.

4. Chicken and Quinoa Salad with Greek Yogurt Dressing

Ingredients:

Grilled chicken breast

Quinoa

Mixed salad greens

Cherry tomatoes

Cucumber

Greek yogurt

Lemon juice

Dill

Instructions:

Grill chicken until fully cooked.

Cook quinoa according to package instructions.

Assemble a salad with mixed greens, cherry tomatoes, and cucumber.

Slice grilled chicken and place on top.

Mix Greek yogurt with lemon juice and dill for dressing.

5. Egg Salad Sandwich on Whole Wheat Bread

Ingredients:

Hard-boiled eggs

Greek yogurt

Dijon mustard

Celery

Whole wheat bread

Instructions:

Chop hard-boiled eggs and mix with Greek yogurt, Dijon mustard, and diced celery.

Spread the egg salad on whole wheat bread.

Assemble sandwiches.

6. Tofu and Vegetable Skewers with Quinoa

Ingredients:

Extra-firm tofu

Bell peppers (various colors)

Red onion

Cherry tomatoes

Quinoa

Instructions:

Press and cube tofu.

Thread tofu and vegetables onto skewers.

Grill until tofu is lightly browned.

Cook quinoa according to package instructions.

Serve tofu and vegetable skewers over quinoa.

7. Shrimp and Vegetable Stir-Fry with Brown Rice

Ingredients:

Shrimp, peeled and deveined

Mixed stir-fry vegetables (snap peas, carrots, bell peppers)

Low-sodium teriyaki sauce

Brown rice

Instructions:

Stir-fry shrimp and vegetables in a pan.

Add low-sodium teriyaki sauce and cook until shrimp are pink.

Cook brown rice according to package instructions.

Serve shrimp stir-fry over cooked brown rice.

8. Quinoa and Chickpea Salad with Lemon Vinaigrette

Ingredients:

Quinoa

Chickpeas (canned, drained)

Cucumber

Cherry tomatoes

Feta cheese

Olive oil

Lemon juice

Fresh parsley

Instructions:

Cook quinoa according to package instructions.

Combine quinoa with chickpeas, diced cucumber, halved cherry tomatoes, and crumbled feta.

Mix olive oil, lemon juice, and fresh parsley for dressing.

Toss salad with the dressing.

9. Chicken and Vegetable Wrap with Whole Wheat Tortilla

Ingredients:

Grilled chicken strips

Mixed salad greens

Cherry tomatoes

Hummus

Whole wheat tortillas

Instructions:

Lay out whole wheat tortillas.

Spread hummus on each tortilla.

Add grilled chicken strips, mixed salad greens, and cherry tomatoes.

Roll up the tortillas to create wraps.

10. Vegetable and Chicken Broth with Rice Noodles

Ingredients:

Chicken broth (low-sodium)

Rice noodles

Chicken breast, shredded

Bok choy

Carrots

Ginger

Soy sauce (low-sodium)

Instructions:

Bring chicken broth to a simmer.

Add rice noodles and cook until tender.

Add shredded chicken, sliced bok choy, julienned carrots, and ginger.

Season with low-sodium soy sauce.

Serve warm.

Dinner

1. Lemon Herb Baked Salmon with Quinoa and Steamed Vegetables

Ingredients:

Salmon fillets

Lemon

Fresh herbs (rosemary, thyme, parsley)

Quinoa

Mixed vegetables (carrots, green beans, zucchini)

61

Instructions:

Preheat the oven to 375°F (190°C).

Marinate salmon with lemon juice, chopped herbs, salt, and pepper.

Bake salmon for 15-20 minutes.

Prepare quinoa according to package instructions.

Steam mixed vegetables until tender.

Serve salmon over quinoa with steamed vegetables on the side.

2. Chicken Stir-Fry with Brown Rice

Ingredients:

Chicken breast, sliced

Brown rice

Broccoli florets

Bell peppers (various colors)

Low-sodium soy sauce

Ginger

Garlic

Olive oil

Instructions:

Cook brown rice according to package instructions.

Stir-fry chicken in olive oil with minced ginger and garlic.

Add broccoli and bell peppers, cook until vegetables are tender.

Pour in low-sodium soy sauce and stir until well combined.

Serve the chicken stir-fry over cooked brown rice.

3. Mediterranean Turkey Burgers with Greek Salad

Ingredients:

Ground turkey

Whole wheat burger buns

Greek salad ingredients (cucumber, cherry tomatoes, red onion, feta)

Olive oil

Oregano

Garlic powder

Instructions:

Combine ground turkey with oregano, garlic powder, and salt.

Form into patties and grill until cooked through.

Assemble burgers with whole wheat buns.

Prepare a Greek salad with diced cucumber, cherry tomatoes, red onion, and crumbled feta.

Drizzle olive oil over the salad.

Serve turkey burgers with a side of Greek salad.

4. Lentil and Vegetable Stew

Ingredients:

Dry lentils

Carrots

Celery

Onion

Low-sodium vegetable broth

Garlic

Bay leaves

Instructions:

Rinse lentils and combine with chopped vegetables in a pot.

Add low-sodium vegetable broth, garlic, and bay leaves.

Bring to a boil, then simmer until lentils are tender.

Serve the lentil and vegetable stew.

5. Grilled Chicken Caesar Salad

Ingredients:

Grilled chicken breast

Romaine lettuce

Cherry tomatoes

Whole wheat croutons

Parmesan cheese

Caesar dressing (low-sodium)

Instructions:

Grill chicken until fully cooked.

Toss together chopped romaine lettuce, cherry tomatoes, croutons, and grilled chicken.

Sprinkle with Parmesan cheese.

Drizzle with low-sodium Caesar dressing.

Serve the grilled chicken Caesar salad.

6. Eggplant and Chickpea Curry with Brown Rice

Ingredients:

Eggplant, diced

Chickpeas (canned, drained)

Brown rice

Tomato sauce

Coconut milk

Curry powder

Turmeric

Cilantro for garnish

Instructions:

Cook brown rice according to package instructions.

Sauté diced eggplant until softened.

Add chickpeas, curry powder, turmeric, tomato sauce, and coconut milk.

Simmer until flavors meld.

Serve over cooked brown rice, garnished with cilantro.

7. Shrimp and Vegetable Skewers with Quinoa Salad

Ingredients:

Shrimp, peeled and deveined

Quinoa

Mixed vegetables (bell peppers, cherry tomatoes)

Olive oil

Lemon juice

Dill for garnish

Instructions:

Cook quinoa according to package instructions.

Thread shrimp and vegetables onto skewers.

Grill until shrimp are pink and vegetables are tender.

Toss cooked quinoa with olive oil and lemon juice.

Serve shrimp and vegetable skewers over quinoa, garnished with dill.

8. Baked Cod with Lemon and Herbs

Ingredients:

Cod fillets

Lemon

Fresh herbs (dill, parsley)

Olive oil

Garlic powder

Black pepper

Instructions:

Preheat the oven to 400°F (200°C).

Place cod fillets on a baking sheet.

Drizzle with olive oil, squeeze lemon juice, and sprinkle with minced garlic, herbs, and black pepper.

Bake for 15-20 minutes or until fish flakes easily.

Serve baked cod with your choice of side vegetables.

9. Quinoa and Black Bean Bowl

Ingredients:

Quinoa

Black beans (canned, drained)

Corn kernels (fresh or frozen)

Avocado, diced

Lime

Cilantro for garnish

Instructions:

Cook quinoa according to package instructions.

In a bowl, combine cooked quinoa with black beans and corn.

Squeeze lime juice over the mixture.

Top with diced avocado and garnish with cilantro.

Serve the quinoa and black bean bowl.

10. Vegetable Omelette with Whole Grain Toast

Ingredients:

Eggs

Mixed vegetables (bell peppers, spinach, tomatoes)

Olive oil

Whole grain bread

Instructions:

Sauté mixed vegetables in olive oil until softened.

Whisk eggs and pour over the vegetables in a pan.

Cook until the eggs are set, then fold into an omelette.

Toast whole grain bread.

Serve the vegetable omelette with whole grain toast.

Snack

1. Berry and Yogurt Parfait:

Ingredients:

Low-fat yogurt

Mixed berries (strawberries, blueberries, raspberries)

Honey (optional)

Instructions:

In a glass or bowl, layer low-fat yogurt with mixed berries.

Repeat the layers.

Drizzle with honey if desired.

Cooking time: 5 minutes (assembly)

2. Vegetable Sticks with Hummus:

Ingredients:

Carrot sticks

Celery sticks

Cucumber slices

Homemade or store-bought low-sodium hummus

Instructions:

Cut vegetables into sticks and slices.

Serve with hummus for dipping.

Cooking time: 5 minutes (preparation)

3. Baked Apple Chips:

Ingredients:

Apples

Cinnamon (optional)

Instructions:

Slice apples thinly.

Place slices on a baking sheet, sprinkle with cinnamon if desired.

Bake in a preheated oven at 200°F (93°C) for 2-3 hours until crispy.

Cooking time: 2-3 hours

4. Greek Yogurt and Fruit Popsicles:

Ingredients:

Greek yogurt

Mixed diced fruits (peaches, kiwi, pineapple)

Popsicle molds

Instructions:

Mix Greek yogurt with diced fruits.

Spoon into popsicle molds and freeze.

Cooking time: 5 minutes (preparation) + freezing time

5. Rice Cake with Avocado:

Ingredients:

Rice cakes

Ripe avocado

Lemon juice

Salt and pepper

Instructions:

Spread mashed avocado on rice cakes.

Sprinkle with lemon juice, salt, and pepper.

Cooking time: 5 minutes (preparation)

6. Cottage Cheese with Pineapple:

Ingredients:

Low-fat cottage cheese

Fresh pineapple chunks

Instructions:

Mix cottage cheese with pineapple chunks.

Serve chilled.

Cooking time: 5 minutes (preparation)

7. Hard-Boiled Egg and Cherry Tomatoes:

Ingredients:

Hard-boiled eggs

Cherry tomatoes

Salt and pepper

Instructions:

Halve hard-boiled eggs and serve with cherry tomatoes.

Sprinkle with salt and pepper.

Cooking time: 10 minutes (boiling eggs)

8. Nut Butter Banana Bites:

Ingredients:

Sliced bananas

Nut butter (almond, peanut, or sunflower seed butter)

Instructions:

Spread nut butter on banana slices.

Create banana sandwiches with nut butter.

Cooking time: 5 minutes (preparation)

9. Caprese Skewers:

Ingredients:

Cherry tomatoes

Fresh mozzarella balls

Basil leaves

Balsamic glaze (optional)

Instructions:

Thread cherry tomatoes, mozzarella balls, and basil leaves onto skewers.

Drizzle with balsamic glaze if desired.

Cooking time: 10 minutes (assembly)

10. Oatmeal and Fruit Cookies:

Ingredients:

Rolled oats

Mashed bananas

Diced dried fruits (apricots, raisins)

Cinnamon

Instructions:

Mix rolled oats with mashed bananas, dried fruits, and cinnamon.

Drop spoonfuls onto a baking sheet and bake.

Cooking time: 15 minutes (baking)

CONCLUSION

As we close the pages of this CKD Stage 4 Cookbook tailored for our beloved seniors, we embark on a journey that transcends mere recipes. It's a journey of resilience, nourishment, and empowerment.

Through these carefully crafted culinary companions, we've ventured into the realm of flavorful possibilities designed to harmonize with the unique needs of those navigating Stage 4 Chronic Kidney Disease.

In each recipe, we find not just ingredients but expressions of care, considering the delicate balance that defines renal health. From vibrant salads to comforting soups, every dish is a testament to the belief that wholesome nutrition can be a source of joy and vitality, even in the face of health challenges.

Cooking for CKD Stage 4 is not a constraint but an art, where mindful choices and creative combinations become the brushstrokes of a masterpiece. It's about savoring the textures of life through carefully curated flavors, fostering a connection between the kitchen and well-being.

As we partake in these culinary adventures, let us remember that this cookbook is more than a collection of recipes; it is a celebration of resilience, a nod to the wisdom of age, and a tribute to the unwavering spirit that defines our seniors. May these recipes not only nourish the body but also feed the soul, adding a dash of warmth and a sprinkle of joy to each kitchen it graces.

So, let the aroma of these dishes linger, let the memories they create be cherished, and may every bite be a reminder that, in the kitchen of life, we can always craft a feast of flavors that resonate with health, happiness, and the rich tapestry of our shared experiences. Cheers to good food, good company, and the boundless possibilities that lie ahead.